GOD, ME, AND ADHD:

The Journey. The Struggle.
The Awakening.

FRANK LAVERGNE, SR.

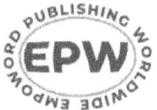

Empoword Publishing Worldwide

17127 Wax Rd Bldg A

Greenwell Springs, LA 70739

www.EmpowordPublishing.com

(225) 317-0593

ISBN: 979-8-714-10411-4

DEDICATION

It has taken me 8 years to find out what I was supposed to write, but I know everything is in God's timing.

This book is dedicated to the amazing and gracious Lord Jesus, that has brought me so far, I can't even recognize myself.

This is also dedicated to the memory of my beloved parents. They did a wonderful job with what they had and what they knew. To impart certain values and principles in me that has carried me into adulthood and that has created a legacy for themselves.

It's a short read because all who deal with this issue lack the attention span for drawn-out long-winded things.

FOREWORD

I believe in divine connection. I believe our Father, who's defined in all his sovereignty assigns certain brothers and sisters to us to connect with, grow with, and learn from for certain seasons of our lives. Pastor Frank Lavergne is a divine connection for me. Without knowing this brother, I knew this brother. There was this divine drawing that led me to this brother in a Smoothie King parking lot.

There was a divine connection that had me ask him to join me on a podcast. There was a divine connection that told me to reach out to him to do an album collectively. This divine leading understood his journey and this path of him being an author. This divine leading knew this moment and ordained it with purpose. Frank is truly a man of God. Those words are often said but rarely confirmed, but he exemplifies that term and the heart behind it. I honor this brother for his yes; his yes, to the calling, to the journey in faith, and the decision to be transparent about his battle with ADHD.

Those yeses will free generations. They will remove strongholds from men and women in faith and not in faith. They will penetrate through the voice of hell and destroy the work of an enemy that speaks lies. They will create a sound that is needed for such a time as this. It is my honor to stand by this brother, and give the foreword for "God, Me and ADHD." You will discover in these pages, what I discovered a year ago, this brother is truly a man after God's own heart.

With Love,
Dr. Ewell O. Netter, Psy.D

Contents

Chapter 1

CHILDHOOD

The signs in childhood

I grew up in the '80s when I think things were pretty normal.

Neighbors would be neighborly, and kids would go outside and play.

There wasn't much crime that I could remember as a child, but things did change as the years would pass by. This new image appeared out of nowhere.

My older peers would go from friends and playmates in the streets to harder demeanors and dark shades. Then they would all hang together at one house and start making money. Then they would use that money and become flashy with cars, clothes, and gold teeth.

Playing with us was no longer fun for them, they would rather make their money and shine. Then school was no longer a priority for them because they were making more money than their teachers.

How my parents raised me I was sheltered from what they knew for a while. I was so oblivious to what they were doing, but I knew they were not the same.

In school, I thought I was ok. But I stayed in trouble and I didn't know why. I was friendly from how I was taught to be. I didn't pick fights and I did my work.

But I was always in the principal's office for misbehaving. The truth is I had both parents and I was scared to death of my dad.

Why I couldn't stay out of trouble was beyond me and my parents. I also known in the neighborhood as Lil bad Frank. But the same way l was at school I was at home. Cool, collected, and a good friend. But people saw me as bad and I never understood why.

So, at some point after all the complaints from teachers and the administration at school. This was around second or third grade I believe, my mom started to bring me to a pediatric clinic to have me checked out. From what I can remember, they told her I was hyperactive and that my brain moved faster than my body.

They also instructed her to limit my sugar intake at school to keep me calm. I would go on to have scheduled check-ups every month or so.

I ended up repeating third grade because of having too many unexcused absences. I felt I had done ok grade wise to pass to the next grade, but the missed days made it an automatic failure.

So, here it is my second go around in third grade and my teacher calls a conference with my parents.

My mom sends my dad because she knew he would get everything cleared up.

As my teacher is addressing my dad about her concerns, suddenly, I hear the words "special ed" the phrase no parent or child would ever want to hear.

This was alarming for both my dad and me. This is around 1992, where I had seen a lot of my friends pulled out of regular classes with me and placed in special ed and to me, all of them seemed normal. None of them looked like they were disabled. Around this time, it was thought that many parents put their children in this situation to get a "crazy check" for them.

But my dad wasn't having it and I didn't want to be teased for being put in special ed. I was already embarrassed about being a grade behind, even though I didn't fail academically. But somehow, I made it through and passed to the fourth grade.

This is when I came face to face with a teacher that didn't play. The school had the authority to spank me and the teacher used it to her advantage. Now, it wasn't abused, but you knew if you got out of line, she would get you, and then your parents would too. She was one who cared and would not let you use excuses. She was hard on us because she knew the world was going to be hard on us.

At some point after getting some help from my mom with my homework. A spark was lit (hyperfocus, we will get to that later) and I could comprehend things now. Everything in school seemed much clearer and it began to show in my grades. To the point, the principal called my mom, because they had built a relationship from all the times my mom had to come up there to see about me and told her "our boy made the honor roll".

So, from the second half of my fourth-grade year to sixth grade, I was an honor roll student. I would amaze my teachers with how fast I would obtain the knowledge that they were given out to the class and how basic I made the curriculum seem. They would tell me how gifted I was and brag about me to their peers.

Then I hit seventh grade and the struggle was real and now that I look back it wasn't the work I struggled with; it was my attention span. I was no longer interested in getting good grades and being a standout.

Plus, other things were going on like girls not wanting the smart guys. They wanted the guy in the back of the class that didn't know anything or acted like he didn't know anything. Also, the smart guys didn't get any respect, they were the butt of all the jokes and the ones getting picked on for being smart and nerdy.

If the cool guys wanted to show off for the girls, it would be the nerds that get pushed around for a good laugh. As for me, I wasn't supposed to be a part of this. I wanted to go to a magnet middle school because I had the brains. I wanted to finish high school and go to college. I wanted a career as an accountant because I was great with numbers and loved math.

But that all took a turn because I didn't want to be clowned and picked on because I was smart. I wanted respect from the cool kids, and I wanted the girls to like me too. I didn't want to be an outcast amongst my peers. So, as you can guess my attention was no longer on books.

Bad enough I was teased for not having what the other kids had, but to be teased for being smart was the straw that broke the camel's back.

So, you see because I was able to hit a switch in fourth grade and achieve, that took the attention off my earlier struggles. So of course, there were no more doctor visits or any more second-guessing if I had issues. I was thought to have had a season of unsureness and then a breakthrough.

Now looking back there were all these signs that I nor my parents could see.

I was now the normal little boy that made them very proud now.

But I was getting less and less interested in school and more interested in being cool.

It started with Easy E and a few other gangster rappers in my ear then come along Master P with the Ice Cream Man. That took my neighborhood and the whole south by storm. Now suddenly, I'm learning how to be street and what a hustler is.

I'm intrigued, I'm learning how not to be lame and what dope is and what weed is. Now I'm smoking cigarettes and weed, drinking beer and liquor. Now I'm starting to get some attention from the girls. Now the big homies that had already switched over started showing me some love. I'm in the zone now, school is all about the girls and recognition. I still did the little work that caught my attention, but it was only to pass time and show the teachers I wasn't dumb. Plus, nobody is going to tease me because I'm bout that now.

My parents never really addressed the change, because I'm still their little boy. I'm just growing and trying to find myself. I'm getting into fights and getting suspended, but it's not my fault it's the kids around me.

They are the ones making me lash out and become defensive. Which was the case, but at some point, I began to enjoy this conflict and would look for it. Because now I've learned how to defend myself well and it's getting me more recognition and respect. So, my parents still have no clue how I'm changing inside because even though I'm starting to get in trouble. I'm still smart and capable of doing good when I put my mind to it, I just got off track.

Now the big one

I get expelled, for possession of marijuana and bullets. I went from smoking to now I'm selling weed at school and I got caught. My parents and everyone but a couple of friends never knew that the day before I had a gun.

So, the following day I'm selling weed but also had gotten bullets from a friend for the gun. I won't go into all the details of the story I made up, but I had my parents and my teachers defending me against being expelled. Because I was able to put on a good show for them while being someone else completely different.

But the campaign that I should not be expelled and continue public school didn't work and I was kicked out. After, the hearing I was assigned to an alternative school for one calendar year and put on unsupervised probation by the juvenile court system.

This is the point I began to hate school. Not only did I miss all the good things that were happening at my old school, but this school was like a prison and they treated us like prisoners. We had to scan through metal detectors and there were no windows. When you checked in you didn't see daylight until you checked out. Even, the meals were like prison food. They would serve us things that didn't make sense, instead of getting waffles and syrup it would be waffles and jelly. It felt like we had messed up as kids and needed to be punished.

I was able to engage the days I did go but that was to make the time go by. Because for some reason in this place the time would move so slow. Other days I would just make an excuse to my parents why I couldn't go or just skip school with some friends. Now the end of the year was here, my charges had been dropped and my teachers had come together. I believe they saw the potential I had when I was there, and they decided to pass me with all D's so I could get to the next grade and maybe find myself.

But that wasn't going to work, I just wanted to get to high school to hang with my cousin and see all the stories that he told me about. I started my first day off smoking weed at the bus stop and getting caught smoking a cigarette by the cafeteria. It seemed like from that day I was on the main disciplinary teacher's radar. But I wasn't there to learn, I tried to change my mind, but it just didn't work. So, I only went when I was bored at home and to see what was going on. If nothing was happening, I would jump the back gate and make my way to my cousin's house.

This went on the first year and at some point, this girl that sat next to me in math class started to take an interest in me and we would clown around in the classroom. Soon things got serious and we began long phone conversations and that turned into a relationship.

Eventually, she did become pregnant and the relationship started falling apart, so we parted ways.

But I'm still in a good space in life. I hit some bumps but now I'm turning it around. I'm working and taking care of my daughter. I'm looking like a productive citizen trying to get my life together. But I have this other career I want to pursue as being a rapper.

Chapter 2

ADULTHOOD

Now I'm 18 and accidentally had started writing lyrics with my friends 4 years prior and had tons of material I had been sitting on. Plus, I have access to a studio now where I can learn to put my words to music. Now I have words over music and people say they like it. Oh wow, I think I can do this. I can have the life I never had and always wanted. Now I'm obsessed with rapping and making money.

But, oh wait you can't be a good guy and rap. You have to be a thug and you better be about what you are talking about or people will call you out. So, I get fired from my well-paying job because I'm too tough to be played with and I'm going to make it big rapping anyway.

I was smart enough to go and get unemployment to keep some income flowing.

I'm finally close to making it because I'm hanging with this record label and they say I'm nice. I'm still not making money from rapping but I'm close. Next, unemployment runs out and it's just me, my daughter, and my mom now, dad checked out. So, I know how to sell a Lil dope, let me go score something and flip it. But my money wasn't flipping, so I can only afford food for us to eat. Momma was paying the bills and I'm at least putting food on the table.

Finally, I land another job and the schedule is interfering with me being with the label. Things are popping off and I can't be around because I must feed my family.

Now, something is going on with my mind. I'm out here thugging and I'm thinking about consequences and God, what's really going on?

Friends thinking I'm cracking because I can't shake this feeling of being judged by God for all my wrongdoings. So much so, that I must go and have a conversation with my mom about it, what is this I'm feeling? I'm feeling so much guilt and shame about how I'm living my life and it's gripping and paralyzing. I'm telling my mom who was at the time watching a Christian network, I need prayer.

At that moment she's thrilled and proud to lead me in a prayer of repentance.

So that night at the age of 21, I gave my life to Jesus and it was an instant change in my attitude and behavior. My mom and I both knew it was real and that the Spirit of God had entered my life. I went and threw everything away that had a bad influence on me. All my CDs, all my raps, and all my weed.

From then I began to hunger for the word of God. I was studying day and night and watching every Christian program I could find (hyperfocus) I purchased new music, what people call church music. I taught myself how to pray and worship.

I started going to church anytime the doors would open and got baptized.

I join prayer groups and leadership classes trying to get every nugget of the Word I could. I was on fire for God but after six to eight months I started to get lonely.

It wasn't that God wasn't enough, it was I had always had relationship with a female for so long and this was the longest I had gone without touching a female. So now my mind was on finding a wife.

I mean I'm 21 and I have a child, and at that time her mom was not around. I began to feel alone, and I was on the search for a wife.

First, I began my search in the church, but the church I was attending was huge with hundreds in service and I felt like I was lost in a sea of people. No one knew me at all except my best friend from childhood and the group of men he introduced me to. Plus, you don't want to be looking like the weird guy always scanning the auditorium looking at females. The thing was that the groups and classes for adults were usually gender separate. So that made it hard to get to know any ladies in the church.

I did eventually have a couple of friendships I was feeling out. One was interested in getting to know me and the other was an ex that I was still good friends with. The first went on for some time but kind of got weird and it tapered off. The friendship with my ex was cool but she wasn't really in the headspace I was in and we kind of lost contact.

By this time, I had bought a car from a friend and was paying a small balance on it as he was helping me get some transportation. Then around the same time, another good friend was helping me out on a second job. I took the second job because who doesn't like more money, right?

So, I'm working these two jobs just grinding for my family and to pay off my balance on my car. A couple of months later my second job, my friend that got me the gig started messing with me about this young lady that was a cashier there. He was like, "look man she the one for you. She's nice, carries herself with respect, and a hard worker".

"You should get her phone number and talk to her". I don't remember how everything carried on, but I showed some real immaturity in the situation. But for some reason, she felt like I was worth a shot and approached me. First, to see why I was tripping but also to see if I was serious about being friends. From that point, we began to talk at work and on the phone and the relationship grew. We would hang out; do some shopping and she would help me pick the clothing pieces I needed to purchase.

Fast forward, we got super close and fell in love with each other. With no boundaries set we soon found ourselves in a situation that we wanted to save until marriage. So, this put us on terms that God would not bless and started causing us a lot of drama that threatened the relationship that started beautifully. Even to the point of a miscarriage and the conception of another child that may not have the family structure that's desired by God.

But someway somehow God started to deal with me again. For me to put myself to the side once again and choose Him. I looked at it as mercy and I might not get another chance if I turn Him down. So, here I am trying to rebuild my relationship with

God and get back on the right track. While having a fiancé that's pregnant and not knowing how she felt about the heart change.

I moved out and got my own apartment to protect my decision to go follow God. But at the same time trying to assure her I wasn't going to abandon them and be a deadbeat. Here, I am praying for a healthy baby, praying that at some point she would feel the same way I felt about serving the Lord and walk with me.

Because now, I'm starting to get these feelings from the Lord again, that I was chosen for a purpose. I'm supposed to do something of value and be of the Lord's service. But I had made a whole mess of my life, how can I go talk to anybody else about their life. After quite some time in prayer and renewing my mind I went to my fiancé's apartment and shared my heart. I asked her if she wanted to be right with God like me and be led in a prayer of repentance.

Now the time has passed, and we know the gender of the baby and time is getting close for our son to be born. As we are trying to get some walking and movement in, my fiancé feels that something is wrong. The baby is not moving like he normally does, so taking no chances we head to the hospital.

Only to find out that the placenta was detached, and the baby needs to come out as soon as possible. Here we are and an emergency c-section is needed and it's a month before the due date.

We braced ourselves and prayed for the best. He comes out underweight, yellow from jaundice, and with a head full of hair. He responds nicely to the smack on his bottom from the doctor, then they proceed to clean him up. Then they hand him to me, my beautiful baby boy and I bring him around for his mom to see him. Now he's off to an incubator and his mom is off to recovery.

Later, they would bring him to the room to let us feed and hold him. Soon, after that, it's time to make his name legal and he takes my name as his. With all these wonderful things going on, besides him being premature. I knew it was only right that his mom and I make the covenant of marriage official before we bring him home. She agreed so, I got a minister to marry us with our mothers as witnesses. Nothing fancy at all just straight to the point to honor God and have him cover our household.

Journey of marriage

It felt so good to finally get the burden of irresponsibility off my chest and move towards the things of God. I had the family I had always dreamed of and things were falling into place. Even though it was good it was a little challenging in the spiritual aspect. Because both of us had different upbringings and different views on things.

For me, I was taught outside of the religious context and showed how to pursue God past the pastor and the traditional things. That I can go to God and ask, seek, and knock. That there are deep truths to explore, more than the surface things you get on Sundays and Midweek. It was pressed upon my heart that I was special and was born for a purpose. So, I wanted to run run run and my wife hadn't been exposed to that type of chasing after God. It always felt like I was running and leaving her behind. Because this is how I was wired, I'm a seeker, a researcher, and very ambitious (ADHD). But she was quiet, humble, and shy. Not wanting to be in crowds or the spotlight.

This made us both question at times are we meant for each other. Because even though we had so much in common which is a lot, we were still different in this way. Soon, I felt like God was calling me to serve at the little church in my neighborhood but for a while, my wife didn't go. She didn't like rapid change and she didn't know any of these people I was trying to force her to know.

As God would have it someone she did know went to this church and turns out it's more.

So, she finally came around and started attending with me and getting comfortable. As time progressed the pastor would see I had a call on my life, and he wanted to be obedient and nurture that call. I would be given small tasks to test my faithfulness. Then more leader building tasks would follow until eventually, I became the youth pastor.

This was it for me, I'm finally fulfilling my purpose and leading a group of teenagers to follow God. Also, I'm doing the same thing the pastor and the church used to do for me as a teen. I'm rocking and rolling, and my wife is right there with me the whole way. It seems as if she had found her groove and felt like she was fulfilling her purpose too.

Then here comes the burnout after four years of serving faithfully and loving it. It's now a burden and I dreaded having to do this on Friday nights, drive all the teens home and get up the next morning for work.

I had a solution though; my associate youth pastor and good friend had come a long way in his leadership role, and I figured he would love to take over. I had witnessed him grow from timid while teaching to being able to control every part of the service and maybe I would take a more elevated less stressful role and help my pastor with the adults.

So, I had the burden off my back, and I can now breathe. Adults aren't that hard to deal with and I don't have to play games with them and drive them home.

Next, I took a much-needed break from all of the Friday nights that I had to rush home from work early to get a nap (chronic fatigue) before service if I could and then get home late just to wake up early and go to work.

This was going to be great and I get to learn how to pastor a church by walking side by side with my pastor. But that didn't last long because, my fourth child is on the way and we don't have enough money coming in, so I must get a second job. I mean after all the church is not paying me and now, I must put pastoring on the back burner to feed my family. This goes on for a while struggling to try to make ends meet. Then we get a break by moving in with my mother in law.

Now, we can stop having to stress about bills. I'm able to sort of go and help my pastor again. My wife and I can go out on dates again and take the kids places instead of being stuck in the house. This is all good for a while but now we are cramped, and we need to get our own place again.

We find a place it's nice with plenty of room for the kids. The rent is kind of high (impulse), but we can swing it (not). It's perfect, we are right around the corner from my mother in law and five minutes from the church.

But the stay didn't last long because we are getting strapped for cash all over again. So, now it's time to look for a cheaper place before we end up getting evicted. We moved a couple more times after that until my dad passed away. My mom had been gone for about six years and now I had lost my dad and on top of that my wife and I had to decide what we were going to do with the house that was left to me.

We decided that we should not let it go down but fix it up and move in. The process took some work and money to get it livable for us and after that we made it home for the next three years.

During this time things were pretty good, and money wasn't tight like in times of the past. But this was mainly due to the mortgage being cheap because as you may know or not, a mortgage is always cheaper than rent. Crazy enough with lower bills I would still find a way to mishandle money and not pay certain things. Then turnaround and take that money and buy stuff that was unnecessary (impulse).

There's no reason to even mention what was bought to save me some embarrassment. Just, know it would be mind-boggling stuff out of impulse. Because, I felt I needed it, never had it, or couldn't stop thinking about it. It was always buy buy buy spend spend spend.

A lot of my behavior I would blame on never having things growing up and it was true to a certain extent. I was never dirt poor and my parents did keep food on the table and a roof over my head. But they just couldn't afford to get me the things most of the other kids had. So, going to school in a time that uniforms were not worn I was the kid that stuck out with the no-name brand clothes and shoes. This went on for my entire academic life except for a few occasions (and I mean a few) when my mom could come through for me.

Yes, that was my excuse for my poor money management, and I was sticking to it.

Chapter 3

How does ADHD manifest

The most noticeable symptom of ADHD is hyperactivity.

It may vary with age. You might be able to notice it in preschoolers. ADHD symptoms nearly always show up before middle school.

Kids with hyperactivity may:

Fidget and squirm when seated.

Get up frequently to walk or run around.

Run or climb a lot when it's not appropriate. (In teens this may seem like restlessness.)

Have trouble playing quietly or doing quiet hobbies

Always be "on the go"

Talk excessively

Toddlers and preschoolers with ADHD tend to be constantly in motion, jumping on furniture, and having trouble participating in group activities that call for them to sit still. For instance, they may have a hard time listening to a story.

School-age children have similar habits, but you may notice those less often. They are unable to stay seated, squirm a lot, fidget, or talk a lot.

Hyperactivity can show up as feelings of restlessness in teens and adults. They may also have a hard time doing quiet activities where you sit still.

Inattention

You might not notice it until a child goes to school. In adults, it may be easier to notice at work or in social situations.

The person might procrastinate, not complete tasks like homework or chores, or frequently move from one uncompleted activity to another.

They might also:

Be disorganized

Lack focus

Have a hard time paying attention to details and a tendency to make careless mistakes. Their work might be messy and seem careless.

Have trouble staying on topic while talking, not listening to others, and not following social rules

Be forgetful about daily activities (for example, missing appointments, forgetting to bring lunch)

Be easily distracted by things like trivial noises or events that are usually ignored by others.

Impulsivity

Symptoms of this include:

Impatience

Having a hard time waiting to talk or react

The person might:

Have a hard time waiting for their turn.

Blurt out answers before someone finishes asking them a question.

Frequently interrupt or intrude on others. This often happens so much that it causes problems in social or work settings.

Start conversations at inappropriate times.

Impulsivity can lead to accidents, like knocking over objects or banging into people. Children with ADHD may also do risky things without stopping to think about the consequences. For instance, they may climb and put themselves in danger.

Many of these symptoms happen from time to time in all youngsters. But in children with the disorder, they happen a lot -- at home and school, or when visiting with friends. They also mess with the child's ability to function like other children who are the same age or developmental level.

Adult attention-deficit/hyperactivity disorder (ADHD) is a mental health disorder that includes a combination of persistent problems, such as difficulty paying attention, hyperactivity, and impulsive behavior. Adult ADHD can lead to unstable relationships, poor work or school performance, low self-esteem, and other problems.

Though it's called adult ADHD, symptoms start in early childhood and continue into adulthood. In some cases, ADHD is not recognized or diagnosed until the person is an adult. Adult ADHD symptoms may not be as clear as ADHD symptoms in children. In adults, hyperactivity may decrease, but struggles with impulsiveness, restlessness, and difficulty paying attention may continue.

Treatment for adult ADHD is similar to treatment for childhood ADHD. Adult ADHD treatment includes medications, psychological counseling (psychotherapy), and treatment for any mental health conditions that occur along with ADHD.

Some people with ADHD have fewer symptoms as they age, but some adults continue to have major symptoms that interfere with daily functioning. In adults, the main features of ADHD may include difficulty paying attention, impulsiveness and restlessness.

Symptoms can range from mild to severe.

Many adults with ADHD aren't aware they have it — they just know that everyday tasks can be a challenge. Adults with ADHD may find it difficult to focus and prioritize, leading to missed deadlines and forgotten meetings or social plans. The inability to control impulses can range from impatience waiting in line or driving in traffic to mood swings and outbursts of anger.

Adult ADHD symptoms may include:

Impulsiveness

Disorganization and problems prioritizing

Poor time management skills

Problems focusing on a task

Trouble multitasking

Excessive activity or restlessness

Poor planning

Low frustration tolerance

Frequent mood swings

Problems following through and completing tasks

Hot temper

Trouble coping with stress

What's typical behavior and what's ADHD?

Almost everyone has some symptoms like ADHD at some point in their lives. If your difficulties are recent or occurred only occasionally in the past, you probably don't have ADHD. ADHD is diagnosed only when symptoms are severe enough to cause ongoing problems in more than one area of your life. These persistent and disruptive symptoms can be traced back to early childhood.

Diagnosis of ADHD in adults can be difficult because certain ADHD symptoms are like those caused by other conditions, such as anxiety or mood disorders. And many adults with ADHD also have at least one other mental health condition, such as depression or anxiety.

When to see a doctor

If any of the symptoms listed above continually disrupt your life, talk to your doctor about whether you might have ADHD.

Different types of health care professionals may diagnose and supervise treatment for ADHD. Seek a provider who has training and experience in caring for adults with ADHD.

Causes

While the exact cause of ADHD is not clear, research efforts continue. Factors that may be involved in the development of

ADHD include:

Genetics. ADHD can run in families, and studies indicate that genes may play a role.

Environment. Certain environmental factors also may increase risk, such as lead exposure as a child.

Problems during development. Problems with the central nervous system at key moments in development may play a role.

Risk factors

Risk of ADHD may increase if:

You have blood relatives, such as a parent or sibling, with ADHD or another mental health disorder

Your mother smoked, drank alcohol or used drugs during pregnancy

As a child, you were exposed to environmental toxins — such as lead, found mainly in paint and pipes in older buildings

You were born prematurely

Complications

ADHD can make life difficult for you. ADHD has been linked to:

Poor school or work performance

Unemployment

Financial problems

Trouble with the law

Alcohol or other substance misuse

Frequent car accidents or other accidents

Unstable relationships

Poor physical and mental health

Poor self-image

Suicide attempts

Coexisting conditions

Although ADHD doesn't cause other psychological or developmental problems, other disorders often occur along with

ADHD and make treatment more challenging. These include:

Mood disorders. Many adults with ADHD also have depression, bipolar disorder or another mood disorder. While mood problems aren't necessarily due directly to ADHD, a repeated pattern of failures and frustrations due to ADHD can worsen depression.

Anxiety disorders. Anxiety disorders occur often in adults with ADHD. Anxiety disorders may cause overwhelming worry, nervousness and other symptoms. Anxiety can be made worse by the challenges and setbacks caused by ADHD.

Other psychiatric disorders. Adults with ADHD are at increased risk of other psychiatric disorders, such as personality disorders, intermittent explosive disorder and substance use disorders.

Learning disabilities. Adults with ADHD may score lower on academic testing than would be expected for their age, intelligence and education. Learning disabilities can include problems with understanding and communicating.

Rejection Sensitive Dysphoria

According to: WILLIAM DODSON, M.D., LF-APA

ADDitude Magazine

For people with ADHD or ADD, Rejection Sensitive Dysphoria can mean extreme emotional sensitivity and emotional pain — and it may imitate mood disorders with suicidal ideation and manifest as instantaneous rage at the person responsible for causing the pain.

Rejection sensitive dysphoria (RSD) is extreme emotional sensitivity and pain triggered by the perception that a person has been rejected or criticized by important people in their life. It may also be triggered by a sense of falling short failing to meet their own high standards or others' expectations.

Dysphoria is Greek for "difficult to bear." It's not that people with attention deficit disorder (ADHD or ADD) are wimps, or weak; it's that the emotional response hurts them much more than it does people without the condition. No one likes to be rejected, criticized or fail. For people with RSD, these universal life experiences are much more severe than for neurotypical individuals. They are unbearable, restricting, and highly impairing.

When this emotional response is internalized (and it often is for people with RSD), it can imitate a full, major mood disorder complete with suicidal ideation. The sudden change from feeling perfectly fine to feeling intensely sad that results from RSD is often misdiagnosed as rapid cycling mood disorder.

It can take a long time for physicians to recognize that these symptoms are caused by the sudden emotional changes associated with ADHD and rejection sensitivity, while all other aspects of relating to others seem typical. RSD is, in fact, a common ADHD symptom, particularly in adults.

When this emotional response is externalized, it looks like an impressive, instantaneous rage at the person or situation responsible for causing the pain. In fact, 50% of people who are assigned court-mandated anger-management treatment have previously unrecognized ADHD.

[Self-Test: Could You Have Rejection Sensitive Dysphoria?]

RSD can make adults with ADHD anticipate rejection — even when it is anything but certain. This can make them vigilant about avoiding it, which can be misdiagnosed as social phobia. Social phobia is an intense anticipatory fear that you will embarrass or humiliate yourself in public, or that you will be scrutinized harshly by the outside world.

Rejection sensitivity is hard to tease apart. Often, people can't find the words to describe its pain. They say it's intense, awful, terrible, overwhelming. It is always triggered by the perceived or real loss of approval, love, or respect.

People with ADHD cope with this huge emotional elephant in two main ways, which are not mutually exclusive.

1. They become people pleasers. They scan every person they meet to figure out what that person admires and praises. Then they present that false self to others. Often this becomes such a dominating goal that they forget what they wanted from their own lives. They are too busy making sure other people aren't displeased with them.

2. They stop trying. If there is the slightest possibility that a person might try something new and fail or fall short in front of anyone else, it becomes too painful or too risky to make the effort. These bright, capable people avoid any activities that are anxiety-provoking and end up giving up things like dating, applying for jobs, or speaking up in public (both socially and professionally).

Some people use the pain of RSD to find adaptations and overachieve. They constantly work to be the best at what they do and strive for idealized perfection. Sometimes they are driven to be above reproach. They lead admirable lives, but at what cost?

Chapter 4

ADHD AND BLACK

The stigma behind getting help

Especially, in the black community, we are too proud to ask for help or think that we need to talk to someone. We can be mocked and ridiculed for "so-called sitting on a couch telling our business". That's one thing black parents don't tolerate, "don't tell nobody what goes on in this house". Besides the few that just can't keep anything to themselves, we don't tell our business, no one else's business, and don't get in other people's business.

You can see this played out in the community with the crime. Somebody saw what happened, but they are not telling anything. Some of it can be intimidation, but most times it's taught to us. Which is why crime prevails to this day in our communities.

When it comes to the black community and mental health, we don't address this issue from a loving and honest ear. We dismiss the notion that something could be hindering us or one of our loved one's mentally from being the person we or they want to be. We assume all a person must do is suck it up and just try harder.

We believe that we as a people have been through so much since slavery and still survived, that it shouldn't be anything within ourselves except for physical handicap or complete retardation. Anything else is an excuse, laziness, or just dumb and slow. This is where we must start putting our pride to the side, be better as people and educate ourselves on these issues.

We as a people need to start building support systems for these issues so that we can identify when our children, family, and friends need help and get them help.

Black children

Often, it's our children that suffer from being overlooked. Not only are they overlooked at school, but also at home and this can be devastating. Teachers already have their hands full, with all the other students in the classroom. All these young different personalities in one place and its worst if it's an all-black inner-city school. It's much to deal with. Most of the kids have attitudes, anger issues, short on supplies, and personal problems that spill over into school.

So, with all of this, it's easy for them to just dismiss a child as a troublemaker, less intelligent, or lazy. Because many of the kids are problems, then it's just normal.

So, the child is either held back for not being academically ready for the next grade or after one or two repeats, just socially promoted. Steady pushing the child through school without addressing the root of the problem. Setting him or her up for a life of low wage jobs, poverty level living, and a cycle that will continue.

On the other end, we have the parents that may have had pretty good grades in school. That expects their child to be just as smart as they were or smarter. Putting an expectation on the child, they can't live up to. Soon threats of physical discipline and hobbies being taken away start to be issued. But, because it's not an academic problem things don't get any better.

Then it's very possible to get into emotional trauma that's caused by not know the reason the child is struggling.

Making him or her, go into a depression, because they don't want to disappoint you or their teachers. They want to be normal and make good grades. But, don't know why they can't. No matter how hard they study, they can't retain the information and fail.

This can be devastating to a child's psyche and self-esteem. Putting thoughts in their mind of not being good enough, being worthless, and it not being anything to live for.

Attention deficit hyperactivity disorder (ADHD) and depression can go hand-in-hand. Doctors sometimes call them comorbid or coexisting conditions, meaning you can have both at the same time.

ADHD is a brain disorder that makes it hard to focus on. Children and adults who have it might have trouble finishing tasks, sitting still, or keeping track of things, appointments, or details.

Depression is more than just an occasional case of the blues. It's deep sadness and despair you feel every day for at least 2 weeks at a time. It can make it hard to work, go to school, or sleep.

Up to 30% of children who have ADHD also have a serious mood disorder like depression. And some experts say that more than half of people who have the condition will get treatment for depression at some point in their lives

Appearance

So much of this is driven by keeping up appearances. We refuse to subject ourselves to anything that is going to make us look weak. This I understand and can relate to, it's so much pressure already on us in society, that of course, we wouldn't want an extra-label of being defective put on us.

We already have to fight twice as hard at everything we do, to break the stereotypes that have been placed on us. It's ingrained in us to never show vulnerability and don't let anyone take advantage of us.

We even, most times alter our behavior, speech, hair, clothing, and skin tone to be accepted by society. So much goes into our appearance, sometimes we lose ourselves. Then we have to hear the community calling us sellouts and Uncle Toms.

Navigating through life as a black person is heavy, it's always a consequence to be paid if we slip.

Medical distrust

As a community, the medical world hasn't always had our best interest in mind. There are plenty of horror stories of black people being experimented on, in the name of medicine.

It's sad that as a people we have had to deal with so much, that it stops us from reaching out for the help we need. Just in my life, I can recall stories of people receiving the wrong diagnosis or medicine, and it cost someone their life.

This recognition has centered on the Black population because of the history of adverse treatment of Blacks by the medical system, dating back to slave experimentation and including the Tuskegee Syphilis Study and current evidence of racial disparities in health care.

However, issues such as discrimination that are likely to increase distrust in the Black community may also apply to other disadvantaged minority populations.

Chapter 5

ADHD AND THE CHURCH

Everything is not a demon or can be just simply prayed away. Of course, prayer is our intimate time with God, sharing all our struggles, and asking in faith for our daily needs. But the sad thing is the Church can be more critical and harsher than the world.

Instead of being the place of healing and safety that it should be. It can also be a place where people not operating in the love and heart of God, can hurt and damage a person's faith. Sending them into despair and leave a person with nowhere to turn.

These days as research is becoming more advanced and revealing what's really going on with the brain. It's time for the church to play its part in the support of those that struggle with mental issues.

I believe this is where the church can minister to the whole person. Because, God desires us to be whole, mind, body, and spirit.

The Mind

"And you must love the LORD your God with all your heart, all your soul, all your mind, and all your strength.'"

Mark 12:30 NLT

This is where the enemy deploys all his attacks. The mind is a battlefield, which Joyce Meyer in her book, battlefield of the mind, goes into detail. Also, Paul tells us to take thoughts captive to make them obedient to Christ, 2 Corinthians 10:5.

You can't love, worship, or obey God, without your mind being free. You can't process things physically or spiritually without the mind being able to work as it should.

The thing with the mind is that it is always vulnerable, unlike the body and spirit. The body is the housing of the spirit and another stronger spirit can come in and take over the ship. But, if God's Spirit inhabits a person, that person can no longer be overtaken by an evil spirit. When it comes to the spirit, it is only affected eternally from the decisions the mind makes. So, for instance, the spirit goes to heaven or hell based on the actions of the mind.

"But I see another law at work in me, waging war against the law of my mind and making me a prisoner of the law of sin at work within me."

Romans 7:23 NIV

Chapter 6

Embrace who you are

"For you created my inmost being you knit me together in my mother's womb. I praise you because I am fearfully and wonderfully made; your works are wonderful; I know that full well."

Psalms 139:13-14 NIV

Now looking at me who would think that I was struggling with a mental illness.

I sure didn't believe I had one and would probably want to fight if you said I had one. But all the signs were there, from when I started school. My parents saw them, my teachers saw them, I would notice them myself, but everyone was oblivious to what was going on.

Attention- parents would buy me toys and I would fully be occupied by it until it was no longer interesting and then I would move on to the next thing.

The lack of motivation- to clean my room and keep it organized.

Clumsiness- tripping and falling because I'm not paying attention to where I'm going.

Hyper - not being able to sit still. I would finish my work early and then distract everyone around me because I was bored.

The bad short-term memory- way before I started smoking weed. I would always lose stuff or my train of thought.

As I got older the money management problems. Not being able to keep the money because of impulse buying.

To the untrained eye, these things look like just behavioral problems

Also, how can something be wrong if you are functioning as a normal person?

After all, I kicked my slump at school to become an honor roll student, I was able to drive and work a job. Plus, to top it off, I had gotten married and I'm making progress in my professional career with promotion after promotion.

How can anything mentally be going on with me?

But subconsciously I was questioning some of my own behavior. Like, why do I not have the desire the keep things organized? Sometimes I do, but I just can't keep it going.

Why can't I finish some of the things I start?

But I knew God had made me special and placed some gifts in me that He wanted to use to bring glory to Himself. So even though, I'm finding out that I don't have it all together. I still knew I was born for a purpose and God loved me.

So, this blew my mind, not only did I finally understand what made me tick. I started noticing other people around me and some of them had already been diagnosed and were getting treatment. Better yet, I could now see these symptoms in my children. They had gotten more from me biologically than I thought. As wonderful as they were, they had my shortcomings too.

It's Biological

Now, that my eyes are open, I can see these traits in my children, and you know the jokes that parents make. "See that smartness and perfection in our child, that comes from me and my side. But, see that anger and disfunction, that comes from you and your side". Even, worst is when the parents are not together, kids are made to believe that they are a screwup like the missing parent.

If you are dealing with this issue or any of the other many mental issues that are out there. I'm here to tell you, that you are not a screwup or a mistake. We all have certain things that are not perfect about us. But, that's because of the curse of sin. Sin came into the world and affected everything, the whole original intent of creation.

When God said it was good, it meant it was perfect, but Adam, messed up that perfection for all of us. It's the whole reason things are the way they are, such as deformed births, natural disasters, animals killing humans, humans killing humans, etc. Everything is sin-stained and in need of redemption.

"For the creation was subjected to frustration, not by its own choice, but by the will of the one who subjected it, in hope that the creation itself will be liberated from its bondage to decay and brought into the freedom and glory of the children of God. We know that the whole creation has been groaning as in the pains of childbirth right up to the present time."

Everything that's wrong with us is biological and has been passed to us through our blood. Sin, sickness, and every generational curse.

But, through God's grace and power that is offered through the sacrifice of Christ, we can overcome. Your family and bloodline don't have to determine where you end up in life.

My personal experience

Yes, it is considered a mental illness and yes it can put a damper on your life. But it has an upside to it, that if you can channel the search for dopamine your brain craves. Which is dubbed "Hyper Focus" you can become an expert and genius in whatever you put your mind too.

Hyperfocus is an intense form of mental concentration or visualization that focuses consciousness on a subject, topic, or task. In some individuals, various subjects or topics may also include daydreams, concepts, fiction, imagination, and other objects of the mind. Hyperfocus on a certain subject can cause side-tracking away from assigned or important tasks.

Psychiatrically, it is a symptom of ADHD together with inattention, and it has been proposed as a symptom of other conditions, such as autism spectrum disorder (ASD).

Hyperfocus may bear a relationship to the concept of flow. In some circumstances, both flow and hyperfocus can be an aid to achievement, but in other circumstances or situations, the same focus and behavior could be a liability, distracting from the task at hand. However, unlike hyperfocus, "flow" is often described in more glowing terms, suggesting they are not two sides of the same condition under contrasting circumstance or intellect.

It can have its disadvantages, especially when it kicks in on the wrong thing at the wrong time, causing you to be totally distracted from the task at hand. But also, that could be a detour that was meant for you to take at that moment. Just, understand this, if you love the Lord. He is going to use every part of you, the good and the bad. For the scripture says

"And we know that in all things God works for the good of those who love him, who have been called according to his purpose."

Romans 8:28 NIV

Everything means everything. I consider hyper-focus my superpower. Because I love to research and when I'm in my zone I am being so fulfilled in the amazing amount of knowledge I am taking in. I love to learn and enjoy when I'm able to get lost in information.

I believe even though there may be downsides to the diagnosis. Once you find what works for you, treatment, or no treatment.

God will bless what people consider a mess. People sometimes do see us as a mess, because we can be messy, disorganized, and forgetful.

Just become aware of who God says you are and walk in that freedom. If you need the assistance of a stimulant, use it under your doctor's supervision and don't let anyone speak you to on what they have not walked in. But, only submit to the guidance of the Holy Spirit, that will guide YOU into all truth.

I do and it works for me and God is pleased that I'm continuing to honor Him with my life. It's not for everyone and that's ok too, everyone is different and responds differently and God loves each of us no matter what.

So, keep your head up, embrace who you are, take control of what you can, and let God handle the rest.

Chapter 7

FAMOUS PEOPLE WITH ADHD

Bill Gates

Bill Gates, born in 1955 is the founder of Microsoft, and has a net worth of $103.2 billion. He also chairs the Bill and Melinda Gates Foundation, the world's largest private charitable foundation which has so far donated $35.8 billion to charity. Bill Gates is known to have ADHD. He talks about dropping out of Harvard as he was itching to start Microsoft at the beginning of the personal computer revolution in an interview with This Morning in 2016. He also discusses his constant activity and extremely busy schedule in an interview with Warren Buffet.

Justin Timberlake

Justin Timberlake, born in 1981, is an award-winning American singer and songwriter. He first appeared in two television shows and then rose to prominence in the late 1990s as the leader of the boy band NSYNC. Justin admits to being both ADHD and OCD.

John F Kennedy

John F Kennedy, born in 1917, was the 35th President of the United States who had countless achievements and overcame many political crises. He is known to have had difficulty with concentration throughout his school years and was known as a mediocre student.

Michael Phelps

Michael Phelps, born in 1985, is a legendary sportsman who was diagnosed with ADHD as a child, according to Psychology Today. He had attention difficulties and behavior problems at school. As an adult, he found swimming to be the perfect outlet for his hyperactivity and went on to become a famous gold medalist swimmer and an excellent example of a high achiever with ADHD.

Simone Biles

The superstar American gymnast with four gold medals from Rio, takes medicine for ADHD. "I have ADHD and I have taken medicine for it since I was a kid," Biles tweeted.

Solange Knowles

I was diagnosed with ADD twice. I didn't believe the first doctor who told me, and I had a whole theory that ADD was just something they invented to make you pay for medicine, but then the second doctor told me I had it.

Michele Rodriguez

Actress Michele Rodriguez gained her celebrity with her role on the hit television series Lost. She told Cosmopolitan that she has difficulty focusing when she is alone. Rodriguez is another example of a female celebrity with ADHD.

Channing Tatum

I read so slow. If I have a script, I'm going to read it five times slower than any other actor, but I'll be able to tell you everything in it. It kills me that there are standardized tests geared towards just one kind of child.

Will Smith

Actor and rapper Will Smith wasn't diagnosed with ADHD as a child. However, he was diagnosed as an adult. Michael Jordan

Considered by many to be the greatest basketball player of all time, Michael Jordan also has ADHD. He went on to win six championships and influence young athletes to achieve their highest potential.

Whoopi Goldberg

Actress and comedian Whoopi Goldberg has ADHD. That did not stop her from winning every major acting award, including an Oscar, a Tony and two Golden Globes

Earvin 'Magic' Johnson

Hall of Fame basketball player and entrepreneur Magic Johnson has ADHD. He has achieved many things, including owning franchise restaurants like Starbucks, Burger King and TGI Fridays.

Stevie Wonder

Composer and singer Stevie Wonder refused to let ADHD slow down his musical aspirations. He is one of America's greatest R&B innovators.

Will.i.am

Will.i.am is best known as a leading member of the band The Black-Eyed Peas. He's also an advocate for ADHD, which he credits for helping his creativity in the music industry.

Albert Einstein

Although it can't be proven, many scholars and historians believe that one of the greatest minds of all-time, Albert Einstein, had ADHD. It's known that Einstein struggled in school and had trouble focusing. However, he was still able to give the world many important scientific discoveries.